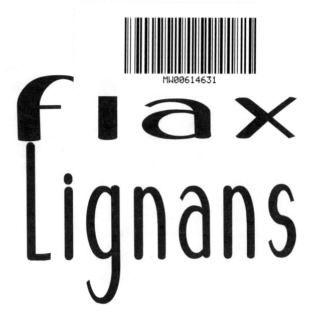

FIFTY YEARS TO HARVEST
Sharing the Inheritance

Irene H. Sönju

and

Beth M. Ley, Ph.D.

(Author of Flax! Fabulous Flax!)

A Health Learning Handbook

BL Publications

Hanover, MN

BL Publications, Hanover, MN
1-877-BOOKS11/www.blpublications.com
email: bley@blpublications.com

Library of Congress Cataloging-in-Publication Data
Sönju, Irene., 1949-
Ley, Beth M., 1964-
    p. cm. -- (A health learning handbook)
Includes bibliographical references
 ISBN 1-890766-37-2
1. Flaxseed lignans in human nutrition. I. Title. II. Series.

Printed in the United States of America

This book is not intended as medical advice. Its purpose is solely educational. Please consult your healthcare professional for all health problems.

Cover design: BL Publications
Cover photos: Courtesy of Flax Lignan Information Bureau
Proofreader: Robin Adams

YOU NEED TO KNOW...
T H E   H E A L T H   M E S S A G E

Do you not know that you are God's temple and that God's Spirit dwells in you? If anyone destroys God's temple, God will destroy him, For God's temple is holy and that temple you are. *1 Cor. 3:16-17*

So, whether you eat or drink, or whatever you do, do all to the glory of God. *1 Cor. 10:31*

Table of Contents

FIFTY YEARS TO HARVEST
Sharing the Inheritance
By Irene H. Sönju
A True Story

PROLOGUE

*The Ukrainian Artist Demetri Farkavec who is known
for painting the smallest work of art in the world has
observed, "The smallest things in the universe are the
most powerful". The hull of the seed of the flax makes
up only l% of a seed; it takes four gallons of seed to
extract out one 5.3 ounce jar of lignans. Scientists are
finding that within the tiny hull of the seed is the
power of SDG (secoisolariciresinol diglycoside) Lignans
in promoting health. SDG is the particular type of lignans flax is especially rich in.*

*It's April 2006. Let me take you back fifty years to
April 11 1955. I was a small girl of five years. All
day I had been waiting for my Daddy to come in from
the fields where he was planting flax seed, to put me
on his lap and sing "Good Night Irene." "That song
was written just for you," he would say. He would then
take the other six and place as many as possible of the
seven of us on his knees as he could to sing "You Are
My Sunshine," give us hugs and kisses and tell us how
beautiful and wonderful we were.*

*That evening, however, as he came into the shed of our
quaint farmhouse, he washed in the laundry tub that
held the rinse water from the clothes Mommy had been
washing on the scrub board by hand all day.*

*I noticed how black with dirt he was, "Potatoes could
grow out of his ears," I thought. That must have come*

from something my Mom had said when we kids, who received a bath just once a week. had gotten too dirty.

Daddy went to bed early that night before the ten o'clock radio news came on. "Mommy come to bed," we heard him call to Mom who was 6 months pregnant with Stephanie, was tucking us into bed up-stairs. The Girls; Margaret 7, Dorothy 6, Irene 5, and Eleanor 3, in one bedroom and the boys; Andy 4, Alfred Junior 2, and the baby Michael 1, in the other.

Something happened that night to cause my Mom to wake us all up after we had been asleep, all except the baby who had been sick with fever all day. She gathered us around her, as she sat in a straight back wooden chair holding Alfred Junior and Eleanor.

The rest of us sat around her on the hard wooden floor in the "hired man's room" up-stairs. She said, "I have something very important to tell each one of you." "Daddy has gone to heaven" and "tonight I'm going to teach all of you how to pray, you will remember this prayer always." "Our Father who art in heaven...." Yes, my Daddy was now in heaven... little did I know that meant he was not coming back.

The farmers that year got together and came with Ford tractors, John Deere's and even a team of horses to finish the planting of flaxseed my Daddy had began so early that year of 1955. We did not harvest those fields as the land was sold within a month of Daddy's death. "It will be better this way" said my uncle to my Mom, because she knew nothing of legal matters.

The land was sold to his friend for $35.00 an acre. We were moved to a small house in town that had

*electricity but no plumbing or running water. Mom
would walk three blocks in the dead of winter to the
town's well in a small park, and hand pump two five-
gallon buckets of water to bring home so we had water
for cooking and bathing. One cold wintry day I went
with Mama to the town pump. She carried two five-gal-
lon, shot-gun buckets filled with water all the way to
the house; a struggle with each step from the weight.
As she reached the steps, she slipped on the ice and
fell, all the water from the buckets spilling out. She
cried, hard. Wiping her eyes, she got a hold of herself,
lifted herself from the frozen snow, took the two pails
and immediately went to the town's hand pump to fill
them again. No, uncles or neighbors were not to be
found. Who could carry the burden of a widow with
eight kids aged eight and under and no twins among
them?*

*Fifty years has passed since the winter of 1956 when
Mama slipped and fell. She went home in December
2005 to be with my Daddy, her years of struggle over.
She carried on through life with her children, her
prayers, and strength that could only be earned
through endurance and love.*

*A few years ago I was called to the same fields my
Daddy planted the spring of his death. I was given a
Promise, whether of my own imagination or otherwise.
"My Daddy's inheritance is mine," along with my brothers and sisters. The fields, the crops, the land that had
been taken from the widow and her children, within a
month of Daddy's death, are now holding monuments
of limestone; great piles of rock stretching to the sky,
perhaps nine great piles, one for each of us, our monuments of remembrance.*

If you go there today, you can still see them. Recently walking the field that day with my son was like walking in heaven because of the soft breeze, the abundant moving waves of grain, and the great mysterious limestone rock piles. The peace was beyond this world. "Your Daddy's inheritance is yours." "Your Daddy is in heaven and you are walking in heaven on this earth." This was the answer to my question of how would we receive my Daddy's inheritance.

Our family is now educating people on the health benefits of flaxseed and flaxseed lignans extract. We realize it has been 50 years to harvest, after my Daddy first planted flax seed there in 1955. After all those years of the seeds of inheritance lying dormant, the harvest is starting to come in. The new research on flax seed as the "healthiest food on the planet" and the invention by our associate of the machine to extract lignans out of the seed have introduced people anew to this food source of which Gandhi said, "Wherever flax seed becomes a regular food item among people, there will be better health."

When our family educates on the benefits of flax and lignans, we are not just offering "the healthiest food on the planet," we are sharing an inheritance which has taken 50 years from seed time to harvest, we are sharing with you our inheritance from the land of North Dakota.

> The scientific name for flaxseeds is
> *Linum usitatissimum*. The meaning of this is
> "*most useful*". This definitely describes the
> versatility and nutritional value of this
> tiny little seed.

Introduction

I was introduced to flax in the late 1980's. Flax quickly became one of my favorite foods. Considering it's tremendous nutritional benefits, I have felt this food has been greatly under-utilized, but things are changing.

Flax is an excellent source of several highly significant nutritional components most people are lacking today: **Omega-3 fatty acids, fiber, lignans and minerals.** Ensuring that your diet contains these offer significant protection against many diseases linked to modern living, including the three major killers of Americans: Heart disease, cancer and strokes.

Blooming fields of flax, found throughout the Upper Midwest (where I grew up) and Canada, are a glorious sight. Flax plants have bright blue flowers topping slender, tough stems. The fibrous stems can be spun into linen and used in making paper and fabrics. The seeds have various industrial uses including the making of paint and linseed oil. The seed, and one particular component of the seed, the lignans, however, in terms of our health, is what this booklet is about.

Flax is nothing new. It is actually one of the world's most ancient cultivated plants. It was cultivated in Babylon 6-7,000 years ago, and has been found among many ancient ruins. The Bible mentions flax at least a dozen times, showing its obvious importance (see Exodus 9:31, Isaiah 19:9, Hosea 2:15, etc.).

Flax was the most important plant fiber in Bible times because it was used to make linen. Clothing was made either of linen or wool. While its production has declined in recent years as cotton is more easily handled by machines, flax remains one of the most important fiber plants in the world.

Worldwide, healers have always believed in the power of flax: Cherokee Indians revered it as a sacred health promoter. Flax seed was consumed in large quantities by the ancient British and Danes. Hippocrates also extolled the health virtues of flax.

Today, much of the world's flax production occurs in Canada and the northern region of the United States where summer days are longer and better for higher levels of Omega-3 essential fatty acid content. The U.S. production is centered in North and South Dakota.

In spite of the long impressive history of flax, only recently has the health industry taken a good close look at flax. Its medicinal benefits are plentiful and its applications numerous.

Flax is rich in fat, protein and dietary fiber. Canadian brown flax averaged 41% fat, 20% protein, 28% fiber, 7.7% moisture and 3.4% ash (the mineral-rich residue left after samples are burned). Composition varies with genetics, soil composition, environment, seed processing and method of analysis.

According to the Canadian Flax Council, the protein content of the seed decreases as the oil content increases. The oil content of flax can be altered through traditional plant breeding methods, and it is affected by geography–the cool nights of northern Canada improve oil content and quality.

The major types of fiber in flax are cellulose (the main structural material of plant cell walls); mucilage gums (becomes very thick when mixed with water or other fluids); and lignin, a highly-branched insoluble fiber

*"Lignin" and "Lignan" are often confused.
Lignin refers to insoluble fiber content.
Lignan is a phytochemical which contains
the hormone-balancing SDG.*

found within the cell walls of woody plants.

Lignins are related to the similar-sounding compound – **lignans**. Both are part of plant cell walls and are associated with cell wall carbohydrates. Lignins, primarily recognized as an insoluble fiber component of flax, contribute to the strength and rigidity of the cell walls.

Lignans are phytochemicals (plant chemicals) whose role in human nutrition, particularly cancer prevention, and the partial list of benefits below, is being actively studied and is the focus of this book.

FLAXSEED LIGNANS BENEFITS INCLUDE:

- Balance hormone health (PMS, Menopause)
- Anti-carcinogenic (fights off cancer)
- Protect prostate health (protect and fight cancer)
- Protect breast health
- Promote regularity- Constipation/diarrhea relief -
- Improve digestion
- Anti-fungal, anti-viral, and anti-parasitical agent
- Improve hormonal skin conditions, such as acne.
- Aid against hair loss (alopecia)
- Reduce elevated cholesterol levels
- Protect against coronary heart disease
- Protect against Type II diabetes
- Benefit weight problems and obesity
- Protect against ulcerative colitis and crohn's disease, irritable bowel syndrome, etc.
- Protect against uterine cancer
- Protect against colon cancer
- Improve sleep patterns
- Provide immune support

Nutritional Facts

Despite the fact that in general, most Americans eat too much, most Americans are **deficient** in numerous essential nutrients. A diet high in refined foods has essentially eliminated essential fatty acids, especially Omega-3s, from our food chain. Also greatly diminished are fiber and minerals. All are greatly diminished or completely lost in processing. These nutrients are ESSENTIAL for our good health.

In addition to Omega-3 fatty acids, fiber and minerals, flax seeds are rich in another very important nutritional components otherwise hard to find in such concentrated levels: lignans.

Other nutrients in flax seed include Omega-3 fatty acids, Vitamin E, beta carotene, calcium, magnesium, manganese, potassium and lecithin. Flax seeds also contain high quality complete protein, providing all essential amino acids.

For more information on the benefits of flax in general, see "*Flax! Fabulous Flax!*" by Beth M. Ley, Ph.D. (BL Publications)

Lignans are found in most fiber-rich plants, including grains such as wheat, barley and oats; legumes such as beans, lentils and soybeans; and vegetables such as garlic, asparagus, broccoli and carrots Flax by far contains the highest level of lignans. Flax contains 0.82–10.55 mg SDG lignans per gram of flax.

Check out the tables on the next two pages for a flax nutritional overview and a comparison of lignan content of foods.

Nutritional Profile of Ground Flax Seeds

Two tablespoons whole ground flaxseed provides:
(One serving = 25 grams)

Alpha Linolenic Acid (Omega-3) . . . . . 1,710 mg.
Linoleic Acid (Omega-6) . . . . 480 mg.
Oleic Acid (Omega-9) . . . . 540 mg.
Lignin Fiber . . . . 1,003 mg.
Lignans. . . . . 13.6 mg.
Calories 140
Calories from fat 90
Total fat . . . . 10 grams
    Saturated fat . . . . 1 gram
Cholesterol . . . . 0 grams
Sodium . . . . 5 mg.
Potassium . . . . 330 mg.
Total Carbohydrates . . . . 7 grams
    Dietary fiber . . . . 5 grams
    Sugar . . . . 0 grams
Protein . . . . 5 grams

Nutritional Profile of Flax Lignan Hulls

1/2 tablespoon of flax hull lignans provides:
(One serving = 5 grams)

Total fat. 0
Lignin Fiber . . . . up to150 mg.
Lignans . . . . 350 mg.
Calories. 20
Calories from fat 0
Total fat. . . . . 0 grams
    Saturated fat. . . . . 0 grams
    Cholesterol. . . . . 0 grams
Sodium. . . . . 0 mg.
Total carbohydrates. . . . . 3 grams
Total fiber. . . . . 3 grams
Sugar. . . . . 0 grams
Protein. . . . . 1 gram

Lignan Content of Selected Foods

Food	Serving	Total Lignans
Flax seeds	1 oz.	85.5 mg.
Sesame seeds	1 oz.	11.2 mg.
Curly kale	1/2 cup, chopped	0.8 mg.
Broccoli	1/2 cup, chopped	0.6 mg.
Apricots	1/2 cup, sliced	0.4 mg.
Cabbage	1/2 cup, chopped	0.3 mg.
Brussels sprouts	1/2 cup, chopped	0.3 mg.
Strawberries	1/2 cup	0.2 mg.
Tofu	4 oz.	0.2 mg.
Dark rye bread	1 slice	0.1 mg.

Source: Milder IE, et al; Lignan contents of Dutch plant foods: a database including lariciresinol, pinoresinol, secoisolariciresinol and matairesinol. Br J Nutr. 2005;93(3):393-402.

Seed Oil (Per 100 gram dry weight)
Flaxseed   370,000 mg.
Caraway seed 221 mg.

Berries
Strawberry 1,500 mg.
Cranberry 1,054 mg.
Red raspberry 139 mg.

Grains & Cereals
Barley 58 mg.
Rye 47 mg.
Oats 13 mg.

Fruits
Banana 3,040 mg.
Guava 700 mg.
Cantaloupe 184 mg.

Legumes
Soybean 273 mg.
Kidney bean 153 mg.
Peanuts 298 mg.

Vegetables
Broccoli 414 mg.
Garlic 379 mg.
Carrot 192 mg.

Flax seeds are by far the richest source of cancer-fighting plant lignans!

Source: Adapted from Mazur W. Bailliere's Clin Endocrin Metab. (1998). Vol. 12; pp. 729–42.

Two researchers at Agriculture and Agri-Food Canada reported that whole seed and ground flax typically contain between 0.7 and 1.9% SDG. This is about 77–209 mg. SDG/tbsp. of whole seed or 56–152 mg. SDG/tbsp. of ground flax.

As you can see by examining the chart on the previous page, flax provides over 100 times the lignan levels other lignan sources do.

Definition of Flax Components:

Phenolic Acids: Phenolic acids are among the phytochemicals (plant chemicals) found abundantly in plants. They appear to have antioxidant, anticancer and antimicrobial activities (Oomah). Flax contains about 8 to 10 grams of total phenolic acids per kilogram (kg) of flax (Oomah). Some phenolic acids could play a role in the health benefits attributed to flax fiber (Harris).

Lignans: Plant lignans are phenolic compounds (Harris). They are biologically active phytochemicals with apparent anticancer and antioxidant potential. Flax is a particularly rich source of a lignan called secoisolariciresinol diglycoside (SDG).

Flavonoids: Flavonoids are polyphenol antioxidants found in many fruits, vegetables and beverages such as wine and tea. These antioxidants bind certain metals, interact with enzymes and have anti-inflammatory actions (Nielsen). Flax contains about 35–70 mg. of flavonoids/100 grams (Oomah).

Antioxidants: Free radical scavanging nutrients (electron donors) that are known to fight cancer and numerous age-related diseases.

SDG Lignans

Lignan-rich foods are part of a healthy dietary pattern, but we are just now beginning to understand the role of lignans in the prevention of hormone-associated cancers, osteoporosis and cardiovascular diseases.

Lignan precursors that have been identified in the human diet include pinoresinol, lariciresinol, seco-isolariciresinol, matairesinol, and others. Secoisolariciresinol and matairesinol were among the first lignan precursors identified in the human diet and are therefore, the most extensively studied. While most research on phytoestrogen-rich diets has focused on soy isoflavones, lignans are the principal source of dietary phytoestrogens in typical Western diets.

Flax is particularly rich in the plant lignan **secoisolariciresinol diglycoside (SDG)**, and it also contains small amounts of the lignans matairesinol, pinoresinol and isolariciresinol.

SDG is converted by bacteria in the colon of humans and other animals to mammalian lignans, enterodiol and enterolactone. Because enterodiol and enterolactone can mimic some of the effects of estrogens, their plant-derived precursors are classified as phytoestrogens. Enterodiol and enterolactone have weak estrogenic activity but may also exert biological effects through nonestrogenic mechanisms.

Mammalian lignans or phytoestrogens work by binding to estrogen receptors on our cell membranes, much like the body's own steroid estrogens do. By doing so lignan phytoestrogens mimic estrogen in the body and can be used as an alternative to Hormone Replacement Therapy.

Increased phytoestrogens have the potential to lower breast and colon cancer risk. Recent research indicates that lignans may be able capable of inhibiting the formation of tumors. Consistent use of flax seed lignans has the ability to increase bowel function up to 30%. Constipation and colon cancer (among other health problems) are also improved.

The significant ability of SDG lignans to prevent cancer is recognized by the National Cancer Institute. In addition to having anti-cancer properties SDG lignans also have anti-viral, anti-bacterial and anti-fungal properties.

Flax seed lignans also have a substantial amount of solid research demonstrating cholesterol-lowering ability. Flaxmeal added to muffins has been shown to lower total cholesterol by as much as 27%. The fiber binds with cholesterol-rich bile acids and carries them out of the body. (Cunnane)

In addition, lignans have antioxidants that help to keep the sensitive oils in the seed from oxidizing before and after it's been eaten.

Mammalian Lignan Production from Foods (Thompson, 1991)	
Food Group (Wet Basis)	**Lignan Content** (ug/100 g)
Flaxseed meal - defatted	67,541
Flaxseed flour	52,679
Dried seaweeds	653 - 1,147
Other oil seeds	161 - 1,130
Legumes (including soy)	201 - 1,287
Cereal brans	181 - 651
Cereals	115 - 651
Vegetables	21 - 407
Fruits	35 - 181

How Mammalian Lignans (Phytoestrogens) Work

Lignans are one of the two major classes of phyto-estrogens (the other class is the isoflavones). They are called phytoestrogens because they are plant (phyto) chemicals that can have estrogen-like actions in human and animal cells when consumed. Enterodiol and enterolactone can mimic some of the effects of estrogens in the body.

Many plants contain chemicals that have estrogen-like actions in animals and humans. These include isoflavones, coumestans, flavonoids, phytosterols and lignans. Lignans are widely distributed in the plant kingdom and appear to play a role in plant growth and in defense against predators (Dinkova-Kostova).

Because the study of estrogen-like chemicals in plants is fairly new, there has been a tendency to apply the term "phytoestrogens" broadly. The criteria to be labeled a phytoestrogen include actions such as whether a plant chemical binds to the estrogen receptor on cell membranes and whether it affects the tissues of humans and animals.

Mammalian lignans are derived from plant lignans. Following ingestion, through the bacteria present in the intestinal tract, SDG is converted (structurally modified) to the aglycone secoisolariciresinol, which is then metabolized to the mammalian lignans (or phytoestrogens) enterolactone and enterodiol. Most of the effects of oral SDG are mediated by enterolactone and enterodiol.

These plant estrogens enter the blood stream and provide a beneficial "buffering effect" on estrogen metabolism. They bind to estrogen receptors in the cells and produce estrogen-like effects that influence hormone production, metabolism, and biological activity. This provides valuable protection against several types of cancer, particularly of the breast, colon and prostate. (Aldercreutz, Ingram, Richard)

A healthy digestive tract helps provide the most benefits of lignans because the type and level of intestinal flora present will affect the SDG production. For example, if you are taking/have taken or frequently take antibiotics, this may greatly interfere with your ability to convert lignans into phytoestrogens. Antibiotics compromise (nice way of saying "kill off") the needed friendly bacteria in the digestive tract.

Therefore, consider supplementing probiotics (acidophilus and bifidus, etc.) and/or eating yogurt or other cultured foods to enhance your ability to use the lignans optimally. Suggestion: Eat your flax lignans with a serving of yogurt (with live cultures).

Because of this detrimental effect resulting from antibiotic use I investigated the possible increased risk for hormonally-related cancers and antibiotic use. I did find several articles, one recently published in the highly prestigious *Journal of the American Medical Association.* (Velicer)

ATTENTION: ANTIBIOTIC USERS

Researchers from Seattle, WA and from the National Cancer Institute in Washington, D.C., looked at medical and pharmacy records of women enrolled in a large health plan in Washington State. The records showed all the prescriptions the women had filled over a 20-year period. They also showed what diseases the women had been treated for, including breast cancer.

The researchers found that the more antibiotics women used, the greater their breast cancer risk was. Over an average 17-year period, women who took antibiotics for more than 500 days, or had more than 25 antibiotic prescriptions, had more than twice the risk of breast cancer as women who had not taken any antibiotics. (Velicer)

For more information visit: http://www.breast-cancer.org/research_antibiotics.html

Lignans and the Sex Hormones: Estrogens and Testosterone

Estrogens are female sex hormones. The primary estrogens are estradiol and estrone. Testosterone is primarily a male sex hormone. The estrogens and testosterone are steroid hormones made from cholesterol by the sex organs and to a lesser extent by the adrenal gland. These sex hormones can be found in both men and women, although the relative amounts differ–men produce considerably more testosterone than estrogens, whereas women produce more estrogens than testosterone. The estrogens and testosterone are responsible for the development of adult sexual characteristics and may influence cancer processes.

The risk of prostate cancer increases as the men's blood level of testosterone increases and breast cancer risk has been linked with higher estrogen levels. (Wynder)

Mammalian lignans (enterodiol and enterolactone) work by binding to estrogen receptors on cell membranes, much like the body's own steroid estrogens do. The bound mammalian lignans affect the receptors' actions within the cell and ultimately the response of tissues like those of the reproductive tract. Other phytoestrogens work in the same way. The mammalian lignans are not as powerful as the body's own estrogens (called endogenous estrogens). Even so, they can act as either phytoestrogens or estrogen antagonists, depending on the presence of stronger estrogens like estradiol. (Hutchins)

Estrogen antagonists oppose the actions of endogenous estrogens. When blood levels of the endogenous estrogens are normal (as in premenopausal women) the lignans can bind to the estrogen receptor and block the actions of endogenous estrogens. In this case, they act as antagonists. After menopause, the levels of endogenous estrogens in the blood decrease naturally because the ovaries release less natural estrogens. In this case, the lignans act like weak estrogens.

Enterodiol and enterolactone may protect against certain cancers, particularly hormone-sensitive cancers such as those of the breast, endometrium and prostate, by interfering with sex hormone metabolism. Lignans may also dampen inflammatory reactions by blocking the release of platelet-activating factor (PAF).

General actions of SDG lignans include:

1. SDG is an antioxidant. It scavenges for certain free radicals (damaging homeless electrons) like the hydroxyl ion ($\cdot$OH). (Prasad) Our bodies produce free radicals continually as we use (oxidize) fats, proteins, alcohol and some carbohydrates for energy. Free radicals (and especially excessive amounts of them) can damage tissues and have been implicated in the pathology of many diseases like atherosclerosis, cancer,

20

diabetes, neuropathy and its many other complications, and Alzheimer's disease. (Praticò)

The flax lignan secoisolariciresinol (Seco) and the mammalian lignans, enterodiol and enterolactone, also act as antioxidants. (Kitts) The antioxidant action of Seco and enterodiol is more powerful than vitamin E, about 5 times more. (Bhathena)

2. Flax consumption doubled the serum enterolactone concentration in 80 volunteers who consumed a combination of ground flax and flax oil in their diets for four months. Increased plasma lignan concentrations were also reported in nine healthy young women (Nesbitt) and in 23 healthy postmenopausal women (Morton) who ate ground flax.

3. Flax consumption increases the excretion of mammalian lignans (enterodiol and enterolactone). Male and female volunteers in three studies consumed 5 - 13.5 grams of ground flax daily for six to seven weeks. Excretion of the mammalian lignans increased 3 to 285-times after flax consumption. (Lampe, Hutchins, Shultz)

4. Flax consumption increases the excretion of estrone metabolites which may protect against breast cancer. In 28 postmenopausal women, consumption of 10 grams of ground flax daily for seven weeks increased significantly the urinary excretion of 2-hydroxyestrogen, a metabolite of estrone that may protect against breast cancer. (Haggans)

5. Lignans bind to estrogen receptors on sex hormone-binding globulin (SHBG), thus blocking

the binding of estrogen and testosterone. As SHBG is found in breast cancer cells, the binding of mammalian lignans to SHBG may interfere with cancer processes that are controlled by estrogen.

6. Pregnant females should avoid <u>overexposure</u> to lignans. Pregnant females and their young offspring are especially sensitive to hormones. While high estrogen levels are needed by the mother to prepare the uterus for the growing fetus, too much estrogen in pregnant animals can reduce litter size and the birth weight of offspring.

Lignans and other phytoestrogens like those in soy, alfalfa and clover can affect the reproductive tract of animals. In rats, exposure to flax diets during pregnancy and lactation had an adverse effect on the weights of sex organs, serum levels of sex hormones, the onset of puberty and, in females, the length of the estrous cycle.

Characteristic for phytoestrogens, lignans can weakly bind to estrogen receptors. A sufficient level of these lignans can compete with natural estrogen for the estrogen receptors, resulting in balanced estrogen levels in the blood.

This by no means is an indication that pregnant women cannot eat flax, it does suggest that large amounts, especially therapeutic amounts, should be avoided. My suggestion if you are pregnant is to avoid the lignan isolate, but go ahead and consume moderate (1 teaspoon) amount of ground flax. It's very nutritional and contains Omega-3 oils needed for the baby's brain development.

One pregnant woman reported that adding a spoonful of ground flax seeds to her diet reduced edema (swelling) in her extremities. (See http://www.babycenter.com/refcap/pregnancy/prenatalhealth/230.html)

Effects in Women

As phytoestrogens, lignans are scientifically indicated to affect hormone levels in women resulting in relief of menopausal problems, improve bone health and support healthy cholesterol levels. In menopause decreasing and fluctuating estrogen levels lead to symptoms such as hot flushes and insomnia. Flax lignans help balance these levels.

Flaxseed lignans can promote normal ovulation and extend the second, progesterone-dominant half of the cycle. The benefits of these effects are manifold. For women trying to become pregnant, consistent ovulation significantly improves their chances of conception.

For women between the ages of 35 and 55 who are experiencing peri-menopausal symptoms such as irregular menstrual cycles, breast cysts, headaches, sleep difficulties, fluid retention, anxiety, irritability, mood swings, weight gain, lowered sex drive, brain fog, fibroid tumors, and heavy bleeding, a probable cause of all these problems is estrogen dominance. Typically, during the 10 years preceding the cessation of periods at midlife, estrogen levels fluctuate while progesterone levels steadily decline.

Flaxseed, by promoting normal ovulation and lengthening the second half of the menstrual cycle, in which progesterone is the dominant hormone, helps restore hormonal balance.

Preliminary research also suggests that flaxseeds may serve a role in protecting post-menopausal woman from cardiovascular disease. In a recent double-blind randomized study, flaxseeds reduced total cholesterol levels in the blood of postmenopausal women who were not on hormone replacement therapy by an average of

23

6%. Lastly, lignan-rich fiber has also been shown to decrease insulin resistance, which, in turn, reduces bio-available estrogen, which also lessens breast cancer risk. And, as insulin resistance is an early warning sign for type 2 diabetes, flaxseed may also provide protection against this disease.

In 18 premenopausal women with normal menstrual cycles, eating 10 grams of flax daily for four months lengthened the luteal phase of the women's menstrual cycle (Phipps). Flax was as effective as hormone replacement therapy (0.625 mg conjugated estrogens) in reducing menopause symptoms among 25 menopausal women who ate 40 grams of ground flax daily for four months. (Lemay)

Effects in Men

Flax consumption does not appear to affect sex hormone metabolism in men. Eating 13.5 grams ground flax daily for six weeks had no effect on testosterone, free testosterone or sex-hormone-binding globulin in six healthy young men. Long-term flax effects of flax consumption are unknown.

By interacting with the complex mechanism of testosterone metabolism, lignans bring back the natural balance in hormone levels such as BPH, a common problem among aging men leading to painful and difficult urination. Other supplements currently sold for prostate bring relief based on anti-inflammatory actions. Flax lignans not only reduce the inconveniences related to urinary flow, frequency and volume, but also decrease the size of the enlarged prostate itself.

Hormone Balancing Benefits

Hormone fluctuations and imbalances associated with menopause, hysterectomy or other reasons had led many to consider the option of Hormone Replacement Therapy (HRT). This very controversial therapy comes with possible negative side effects and risks. Animal estrogen (from HRT) can increase risk for uterine cancer. Progesterone, the other component of HRT, reduces the risk of uterine cancer, but increases the chance of breast cancer.

The best and natural alternative is to eat foods high in plant estrogens. Recent studies have also shown both soy products and flax seeds to be promising in the blocking of male and female hormone-related cancers, such as breast, colon, rectal and prostate. Studies also indicate that the health benefits of eating flax may be cumulative. (Wang, Lei, Hong, Stattin)

Flax is Safe Alternative to HRT

Flax seed lignans can be an alternative or supplement to HRT. Isoflavones help relieve hot flashes, night sweats, lowers cholesterol, safeguards heart and bone health, promotes vaginal moisture and have almost no negative effects.

Researchers at the Department of Food Science and Nutrition, University of Minnesota, St. Paul, reported on the benefits of flaxseed lignans in postmenopausal women. Dietary estrogens, such as lignans may act to alter hormone metabolism and subsequent cancer risk. Consumption of flax increases excretion of enterodiol and enterolactone. (Hutchins)

Ovarian hormone deficiency is a major risk factor for osteoporosis in postmenopausal women. However, many women are opting against HRT for fear of cancer and other contraindications.

Research led by Bahram Arjmandi, Ph.D., of the Department of Nutritional Sciences at Oklahoma State University, Stillwater, shows that phytoestrogens (as in flax) help prevention and treat osteoporosis in women with ovarian hormone deficiency. (Arjmandi)

In earlier research, Dr. Arjmandi also showed that **ground flax seed lowers cholesterol and reduces a heart disease-promoting protein in postmenopausal women.** In the double-blind, crossover study, 38 women with extremely high cholesterol levels were given bread and muffins containing 38 grams of either sunflower or flax seed flour daily.

Flaxseed lowered total cholesterol by 6.9% (from 229 to 213 mg/l) and LDL cholesterol by 14.7% (from 158 to 133 mg/l). Another study showed a 12% reduction in total cholesterol (from 241-213 mg/l), taking 30 grams ground flax (just over 1/4 cup) daily. (Demark-Wahnefried)

Even more importantly, **flax lowered levels of a protein called lipoprotein(a), or Lp(a)**, from 0.95 to 0.88 mm/l. Lp(a), which increases after menopause, causes atherosclerosis in several ways. It increases clotting and cholesterol deposition in artery walls and oxidizes LDL cholesterol, making it highly reactive. Lp(a) levels are lowered by estrogen supplementation but not by cholesterol-lowering drugs, which may explain estrogen's protective effect on the heart. This study demonstrates the first dietary approach to lowering Lp(a).

Flaxseed is high in Omega-3 fatty acids, known to lower cholesterol, and lignans, which have a weak estrogenic effect on fats. According to Arjmandi, *'The potential effects of flaxseed on lowering blood cholesterol and Lp(a) in postmenopausal women have immense implications should this dietary source of polyunsaturated fatty acid and lignan precursors be demonstrated effective."* (Arjmandi,1998)

Flax Superior to Soy

When discussing phytoestrogens, most people usually think of soy, yet flax is actually a much more potent plant source of estrogen. Flax has an additional advantage over soy in that flax contains no goitrogenic substances that interfere with thyroid functioning.

"there is abundant evidence that some of the particular isoflavones found in soy, including genistein and equol, a metabolite of daidzen, demonstrate toxicity in estrogen sensitive tissues and in the thyroid. This is true for a number of species, including humans.

Additionally, these isoflavones are inhibitors of the thyroid peroxidase which makes the thyroid hormones T3 and T4. Inhibition can be expected to generate thyroid abnormalities, including goiter and autoimmune thyroiditis. There exists a significant body of animal data that demonstrates goitrogenic and even carcinogenic effects of soy products. Moreover, there are significant reports of goitrogenic effects from soy consumption in human infants and adults."

Statement made by Daniel Doerge and Daniel Sheehan, two key experts on soy to the Food and Drug Administration (FDA).

Osteoporosis Benefits

Proper blood levels of estradiol, estrone, and estrone sulfate are important since estradiol is involved in maintaining bone mass. Flax lignan phytoestrogens also exert some degree of protection against the loss of calcium and other minerals and so have been considered of possible benefit in treating osteoporosis, especially for women with ovarian hormone deficiency or postmenopausal women. (Knight) A number of studies show that addition of phytoestrogens to the diets resulted in reduced bone turnover and other markers indicating improved bone density. (Van de Poll)

Cardiovascular Benefits

Antioxidant benefits of SDG protect against free radical damage which contributes to plaque buildup in the arteries. One animal study using flax lignans showed a 73% reduction of atherosclerosis-plaque build-up in the arteries. The lignans also reduced total and LDL (bad) cholesterol. (Prasad)

Healthy Skin

A common benefit to individuals (males and females of all ages) supplementing their diets with high lignan flaxseed oil or ground flax is improvment of acne problems. Hormonal imbalances (often elevated testosterone or other androgens) are a common cause of acne breakouts. Flax lignans have been shown to inhibit 5 alpha reductase, an enzyme involved in the conversion of testosterone to DHT, the more active form of testosterone. Lower levels of DHT is therefore, very helpful.

Many other skin conditions also respond to flaxseed and flax oil supplements; psoriasis, eczema, hives and dry, scaly skin.

Hair Loss

Androgenetic alopecia is the most common type of hair loss in men and women. This is a testosterone dependent process. Studies show a high level of DHT is associated with male pattern baldness, alopecia and possibly other causes (such as stress related) of hair loss as well.

When a hair is shed, DHT initiates the miniaturization of hair root and follicle. Lignans balance DHT levels and thereby prevent hair follicles from being miniaturized.

Other Research of Interest

Researchers also tell us that lignans offer a variety of beneficial protective effects for our health as they are are platelet activating factor (PAF)-receptor antagonists. PAF is a substance released by certain white blood cells (basophils and mast cells) in immediate hypersensitivity reactions and macrophages and neutrophils in other inflammatory reactions that lead to bronchoconstriction (**asthma),** platelet aggregation (clotting), and the release of vasoactive substances from platelets. It is also found to be a contributor in numerous health problems, including allergies, kidney disease, and numerous inflammatory conditions.

Researchers at the University of Western Ontario, London, Canada, investigated the beneficial effects of flax lignans in lupus nephritis patients. They found 30 grams of flax seed per day (slightly over 1/4 cup) benefited kidney function as well as inflammatory and atherogenic mechanisms important in the complications associated with lupus nephritis. (Clark)

Therapeutic Effects of Lignans

Researchers at the Nutrition and Cancer Folkhalsan Research Center, University of Helsinki, Finland, report that phyto-estrogens from lignans have a preventive effect against various cancers, specifically breast, prostate and colon cancer. Several studies have shown that a **low**-lignan diet increased the risk of breast cancer. (Adlercreutz) Other studies show flax caused a decrease in tumor size.

Italian researchers also are investigating the protective role lignans seem to have against liver disease. (Lei)

Breast Cancer

Studies suggest lignans are highly protective against breast cancer. A study in Finland found that women with high levels of enterolactone in their blood had a lower risk of breast cancer. This study and others suggest that a diet high in lignans may be protective against breast cancer. (Pietinen) Flax lignan consumption increases enterolactone levels.

A study at the University of Toronto, Ont, Canada, showed, for the first time, that flax SDG has an anti-tumor effect when provided at the early promotion stage of tumorigenesis. (Thompson)

In a study with postmenopausal women, those consuming flax had a protective effect against breast cancer. Amounts consumed were 0, 5, and 10 grams of ground flax seed daily for seven weeks. Those who ate flaxseed had higher levels of estrogen metabolites, again suggesting that flaxseed is protective against breast cancer. The greater the intake of flax, the greater the beneficial effects. (Haggans)

In another study with premenopausal women, 10 grams of ground flax daily showed improvement in the ratio of estrogen metabolites.

Finally, a study with woman with newly diagnosed cancer examined the effects of flax on the cancer growth. They compared the effects of a group of women who ate a daily muffin containing 25 grams of ground flax compared to those eating a muffin with no flax for about one month. They found the woman who ate the flax had reductions in breast cell proliferation and tumor growth and a rate similar to effects seen with tamoxifen (a breast cancer drug treatment). (Thompson)

Similar effects on breast cancer have been seen in animal studies.

Research also suggests that lignans may decrease the blood vessels that feed the tumors. (Dabrosin) Decrease the food source... decrease the tumor.

Flax IS Safe to Use With Tamoxifen

Many women recovering from breast cancer ask me about the safety of using flax or flax lignans with the drug tamoxifen, which is commonly prescribed for breast cancer. Animal studies show that a diet of 10% ground flax seed (that is A LOT of flax!) inhibited the growth of human estrogen-dependent breast cancer and strengthened the tumor-inhibitory effect of tamoxifen. Tumors reduced in size as much as 74% in the flax group. The researchers reported their results as encouraging, providing some scientific justification for the clinical testing of flax seeds in both pre- and postmenopausal breast cancer patients taking tamoxifen. (Chen)

Jianmin Chen, Faculty of Medicine, University of Toronto, reports that tumor regrowth caused by tamoxifen (alone) is a significant problem. Resistance usually occurs after prolonged treatment. (Chen) Use of flax lignans could possibly prevent this. While more research is needed to prove it's degree of effectiveness, we do know that the use of flax in this way is safe.

Prostate Cancer

Cancer of the prostate is the second most commonly diagnosed cancer after skin cancer in the male population of the United States and the second most common cause of death from cancer after that of the lung.

The lignans in flax which convert to the important phytoestrogens enterodiol and enterolactone also serve to protect against prostate cancer. (Evans) The protective effects of lignans may be due to their ability to compete with estrogen receptors, to induce sex hormone binding globulin, to interfere with 5 alpha-reductase isozymes 1 and 2 (Evans) of which high levels are associated with cancerous prostate tissue (Rennie), to inhibit placental aromatase, and to also act as antioxidants. (Wang, Lei, Hong, Stattin, Griffiths, Hedelin)

A Swedish study where individuals ate 30 grams (slightly over 1/4 cup) ground flax daily demonstrated a statistically significant decrease in PSA (8.47 to 5.72 ng/mL) after 6 months. (Demark-Wahnefried)

Diabetes and Blood Sugar Effects

Studies reporting on the effects of lignans on chemically-induced diabetes mellitus in rats show plasma glucose levels were reduced 63% in lignan-treated animals. Flaxseed meal is also rich in a number of other components that may favorably affect glucose metabolism. Bread enriched with 25% flax seed produced a blood glucose response 28% lower than bread containing only wheat flour. Slowly digested foods (such as unrefined whole foods) may prevent the onset of diabetes and improve insulin sensitivity and reduce insulin resistance.

Flax contains mucilage on the outside of the seed coat. Acting as a soluble fiber, mucilage increases the viscosity of the small intestinal contents and delays the digestion and absorption of carbohydrates. Flaxseed protein also may be important in reducing the glycemic response of foods due to its interaction with starch. (Thompson and Cunnane)

Adding ground flax seed to a food with a high glycemic index (such as bread, pancakes, white rice, fruit juice, etc.), reduces the glycemic response of the body. This is an excellent benefit not only for diabetics, but for anyone interested in losing weight or with constipation problems because of the fiber increase.

Flax Lignans Reduce Type I and II Diabetes

Research has suggested that Type I diabetes may be due to oxidative stress (free radical damage). Studies have also already demonstrated effectiveness of SDG isolated from flax seed for Type I. (Prasad, 2000)

Researchers at the University of Saskatchewan, Canada wanted to determine whether Type II diabetes is due free radical damage and whether SDG could prevent the development of diabetes. They administered 40 mg./kg. body weight, orally in drinking water to Zucker diabetic fatty rats, a model of human Type II diabetes.

Incidence of diabetes was 100% in the untreated group but only 20% in the SDG-treated rats by the age of 72 days. The rats that did not develop diabetes by 72 days of age in the SDG-treated group developed diabetes later on (age 72 to 99 days) except for 10% of the rats that did not develop diabetes for the duration of the study (101 days of age).

This suggested that SDG from flax seed retarded the development of diabetes. Diabetes was associated with an increase in oxidative stress indicated by an increase in serum free radicals. Also, diabetes was associated with an increase in serum total cholesterol and triglycerides and glycated hemoglobin A. SDG-treated rats that did not develop diabetes by 70 days of age had no increase in oxidative stress, serum total cholesterol, and glycated hemoglobin. These results suggest that Type II diabetes is associated with an increase in oxidative stress (free radical damage) and that SDG is effective in retarding the development of diabetes. (Prasad, 2001)

In the earlier Type I study, SDG from flax seed prevented the development of diabetes by approximately 71%. Type I diabetes was 72.7% in untreated and 21.4% in SDG-treated group. Prevention in development of diabetes by SDG was associated with a decrease in serum and pancreatic-oxidants (free radicals) and an increase in antioxidant reserves. (Prasad, 2000)

Safety and Side Effects

Flax is extremely safe and free of side effects. Lignans in foods have no known adverse effects. Flax seeds, rich in lignans and fiber, may increase stool frequency or cause diarrhea in high doses (45-50 g/day = about 5 tablespoons). Individuals not accustomed to a diet high in fiber may experience a temporary increase in gas. Avoid this by starting with small amount and gradually increasing the dosage.

The safety of lignan supplements in pregnant or lactating women has not been established. For precautionary reasons, my recommendation is to **avoid lignan isolates** if you are pregnant or lactating, but consuming up to <u>one teaspoon</u> of ground whole flax daily is acceptable -alone or in food (like a piece of flax banana date bread).

Like almonds and cashews, raw flax seeds contain a very small amount of thiocyanate, a toxic cyanide-like compound. This can be found in the blood after eating raw flax seed, but not in quantities significant enough to cause any health problems. There are no reports of toxicity or health problems from this substance.

After eating foods containing thiocyanate, enzymes in the body convert it into a harmless nontoxic form. Cooking also neutralizes this compound, making it completely harmless in any quantity. (Cunnane, Bricklin)

A Finish study demonstrated the safety of consuming a diet high in raw flax meal (20% of total calories). A 2,000-calorie-per-day diet would require almost 3/4 cup of ground flax to provide 400 calories. That is a lot of flax - three times more than the suggested intake of 1/4 cup daily. This resulted in significantly higher amounts of fiber, Omega-3, EPA, DHA and serum enterolactone concentration doubled during flax seed supplementation. Serum thiocyanate and blood cadmium values did not exceed safe reference values and no adverse effects were reported. (Tarpilla)

Flax Lignan Products

Flax seeds should not be consumed whole as they will simply pass through the body (unless you chew each seed thoroughly, which is nearly impossible!). The shell of the seed needs to be broken down by grinding or by soaking in something like buttermilk (which contains live enzymes) to weaken the cell wall. If the shell is not broken down, the healthy contents inside the flax seed cannot be absorbed and used by the body.

Considerations when product shopping:

Ideally, look for **organic and non-GMO (genetically modified)** products.

"Standardized" lignan products are not necessary but will give a better idea of what dosage you are consuming if you desire therapeutic doses.

Lignans Available as Isolate

Commercial methods for extracting and purifying the lignans in flax are now available, thus making it possible to just supplement the lignans, and for food

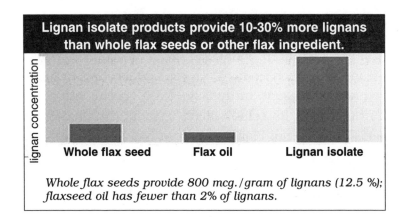

Lignan isolate products provide 10-30% more lignans than whole flax seeds or other flax ingredient.

lignan concentration

Whole flax seed   Flax oil   Lignan isolate

Whole flax seeds provide 800 mcg./gram of lignans (12.5 %); flaxseed oil has fewer than 2% of lignans.

companies to add pure SDG lignans to food products.

NDSU researchers have isolated the lignan component which provides a concentrated lignan product excellent for therapeutic purposes. This form is by far the most concentrated method of obtaining high (therapeutic) amounts of lignans.

Flax oil containing added lignans has been available for several years. One oil product tested contained 0.1% SDG or about 14 mg SDG/tbsp flax oil. The amount of SDG obtained from a lignan-enriched oil depends on how well the SDG particles mix with the oil. Adding SDG to flax oil is a bit like mixing oil and water–because SDG is not soluble in oil, it resists mixing with the oil and tends to settle in the bottom of the container (so be sure to shake it before using). Even if the oil labels says high lignan content, it's levels are minimal even compared to whole flax seed.

Lignan supplements (in the form of capsules) derived from flaxseed are also available in the U.S. One such supplement provides 50 mg of secoisolariciresinol diglycoside (SDG) per capsule.

Flax lignan capsules or powder can be safely used if you are also using ground flax seeds on a regular basis.

How to Use Flax Lignans

Flax has been long-used in multi-grain cereals, breads and snack foods. When you add flax to your food, you add a pleasant, nutty taste, extra texture and good nutrition with its soluble fiber, lignans, Omega-3 fatty acids and protein. Flax lignans can be used similarly to flax seeds, but in much less concentration. A serving of ground flax seeds is from one to two tablespoons. A serving of flax lignans is about 1/2 tablespoon.

If you are using whole seeds instead of lignan isolate products, the flax seeds need to be ground into a flour-like powder (a coffee bean grinder or a blender work great) as you use them. This is done to preserve the fatty acids in flax seed from breaking down and becoming rancid. These fatty acids are highly susceptible to destruction by exposure to heat, light and oxygen. Optimally, use the flax the same day it is ground.

Finely ground your seeds to obtain more benefit from the SDG lignans. Higher yields of SDG result from finely-ground flax compared to coarsely-ground flax. (Muir)

Once the shell of the seed has been broken, the inside elements are exposed and the enzymes and antioxidants that have kept the oils fresh (inside the shell) now rapidly disintegrate. The longer the meal sits before it's eaten, the more oxidation or free-radical damage occurs. *(Note: This does not apply to lignan isolates where the oil has been removed.)*

If you must grind flax in advance, store it in airtight plastic (small zipper-lock bags work well) removing as much air as possible, and wrap tightly in tin foil to keep light out. Store it in the freezer, refrigerator or in a cooler if you are traveling. The lignans remains in tact.

Ground flaxseed (flaxseed meal) or lignans can be

consumed raw or in baked goods such as bread, cookies, pancakes, muffins or cooked dish, casseroles, etc. The fiber and lignan benefits remain through cooking, but some of the essential fatty acid (from ground seeds) will be lost. The higher the temperature, the more destruction of the oil (from the ground seed) will occur.

Flax Daily Dosage:

Ground Whole Seeds:
2 tablespoons (Maintenance)
1 tablespoon = 10 grams flax seed = 50 to 150 mg lignans.
1/4 cup (Therapeutic)

Lignan Isolate:
1/2 tablespoon (5 grams) (Therapeutic)
5 grams = 150 mg. lignans

Suggestions for Lignan Isolate
(Lignan isolate dosage is lower compared to grinding your own whole seeds.)

- ❖ Mix 1/2 tbsp. with a serving of yogurt, cottage cheese, cheese dip, etc.

- ❖ Stir in 1/2 tbsp. with a serving of peanut or almond butter to spread on toast or celery.

- ❖ Add two tablespoons into homemade breads, waffles, pancakes, muffins or other baked goods before baking.

- ❖ Sprinkle 1/2 tbsp. on salads, scrambled eggs, hot or cold cereal, rice or steamed vegetables.

- ❖ Blend into smoothies or fruit shakes (1/2 tbsp. per serving).

- ❖ Stir 1/2 tbsp. into a glass of juice.

- ❖ Add 1/2 tbsp. to soups; tomato. chicken noodle, etc.

Recipes

Oatmeal Flax Muffins *(Plain, raisin, apple or orange)*

    1 1/2 cups old-fashioned rolled oats
    1/4 cup steel cut oats
    1/8 cup flax seeds (whole)
    2 cups fat free buttermilk
    Combine and let these ingredients soak for 1-2 hours
    Add:
    1/2 cup brown sugar *(can also use honey or 1/4 cup brown sugar & 1/4 cup honey)*
    2-3 tbsp. applesauce (optional)
    1 whole egg plus 2 egg whites
    1 1/4 cups whole wheat flour (approx..) *or substitute amaranth, triticale or other whole grain flour*
    1/2 tsp. baking soda
    1 tsp. baking powder
    1/2 tsp. salt
    1/4 cup freshly ground flax seed

Options to add:
    Cinnamon (1 tsp.)
    Cardamom (1/2 tsp.)
    Raisins
    Chopped apple
    Grated orange peel and 1-2 tsp. of frozen orange juice conc.

Pour into muffin tins; bake in 375° oven for 18 minutes. Yield: 12 or 14 muffins
Store extras in the freezer for a quick breakfast or snack!!!

Flax-Almond Whole Wheat Cookies

    1/2 cup whole flax seeds
    1 cup kefir or buttermilk
    1/2 cup butter (room temp.)
    2 cups turbinado (raw) sugar
    2 eggs
    2 tbsp. pure vanilla extract
    2 cups whole wheat flour
    1/2 cup freshly ground flax seeds
    1 tsp. baking soda
    1 tsp. baking powder
    1/2 tsp. sea salt
    1 cup freshly chopped almonds *(or 1 tsp. cardamom and 1/4 tsp. cloves)*

Soak first two ingredients for 2 hours. In a separate bowl, cream butter and turbinado sugar until fluffy. Add one egg at a time and then add vanilla. In another bowl combine flour, ground flax, baking soda, baking powder and salt. Stir in soaked flax seeds and the butter-egg mixture and mix well. Add almonds (or spices). Form dough into balls and place on a cookie sheet 2 inches apart. Bake at 350° for 15 minutes. Remove and cool on a cooling rack.

Flax Oatmeal Cookies

1 cup butter
1 cup turbinado sugar
1 cup brown sugar
2 eggs
1 tsp. vanilla
1/2 cup ground flaxseed
1/2 tsp. salt
1 tsp. baking powder
1 tsp. baking soda
1 tsp. cinnamon
1 cup all-purpose flour
1 cup whole wheat flour
1 1/2 cups old fashioned rolled oats

Cream butter and sugar until light and fluffy, add eggs and vanilla and beat well. Mix together flour, oats, ground flax, salt, baking powder, baking soda and cinnamon. Stir into creamed mixture. Mix until well blended Form into 1-2 inch balls, place on ungreased cookie sheet about 2 1/2 inches apart. Bake at 350° for 10 minutes.

Whole Wheat Flax Bread

1 cup room temperature water
3 tbsp. honey
1 tbsp. olive oil
1 1/2 cups bread flour
1 1/2 cups whole wheat flour
1 tsp. salt
1/2 cup ground flax seeds
2 tsp. fast rising instant yeast
Optional: 1 tbsp. sunflower seeds or 1 tbsp. poppy seeds

Measure ingredients and place in bread machine pan in order recommended by the manufacturer. Select Whole Wheat Rapid Cycle. Remove baked bread from pan. Cool on wire rack.
Note: Try adding about 1/3 cup of ground flax seeds and about 2 tbsp. of honey to any commercial bread mix flavor.

Banana-Date Flax Seed Bread

1 cup ground flax seeds
2/3 cup mashed banana
1/2 cup honey plus 1 tsp. stevia
2 eggs
1 cup whole wheat flour
1/2 cup flax - whole seeds
1 tsp. baking powder and 1 tsp. baking soda
1 tsp. salt
1 cup chopped pitted dates

Beat the banana, honey or stevia and eggs at medium speed until well blended. Combine flour, ground flax seeds, whole flax seeds, baking powder, baking soda and salt. Gradually add to mixture, beating until well-blended. Stir in dates and pour into a greased 8 x 4 inch loaf pan. Bake at 350° for 55 minutes or until a wooden pick inserted comes out clean. Cool 10 minutes in pan and remove. Cool on wire rack.

Granola

>   4 cups old-fashioned rolled oats
>   1/4 cup poppy seed
>   1 1/2 cups wheat germ
>   1 cup sesame seeds
>   1 cup slivered almonds or sunflower seeds
>   1/2 cup whole raw almonds
>   1/2 cup honey or real maple syrup
>   1/3 cup olive oil
>   1/2 cup water
>   1/2 cup flax seed
>   1 cup shredded coconut (optional)
>   1 cup raisins
>   2-3 teaspoons cinnamon

Combine together all dry ingredients into a large bowl. Heat honey, oil, and water until well blended. Add liquid to dry ingredients and mix well until all dry ingredients are moistened. Place on a cookie sheet (or two); bake at 350° F. for 30 minutes. Stir every 10 minutes for even toasting.

Flax Fruit Bars

>   1/3 lb. raisins
>   1/4 lb. dates
>   2 tbsp. raw honey (can add more if mixture does not stick together)
>   1/2 cup ground flax seeds
>   1/4 cup wheat germ
>   1/4 cup shredded coconut

Chop fruit in food processor. Mix in honey, flax, wheat germ and coconut. Mold mixture in a pan and refrigerate 1 hour. Cut into bars and serve. You can wrap bars in plastic wrap for a healthy snack to keep in your purse or backpack.

Berry Berry Smoothie

>   1/2 cup frozen raspberries
>   1/2 cup fresh or frozen strawberries
>   1/4 cup cranberries (or other fruit–blueberries, peaches, chopped apple, etc.)
>   3/4 cup berry juice (more for thinner consistency)
>   1/8 cup protein powder (optional)
>   1 cup plain yogurt
>   1/8 cup ground flax seeds

Mix together in blender. Makes about 2 servings.

Orange Dream Smoothie

>   1 peach, orange or nectarine
>   3/4 cup orange juice (more for thinner consistency)
>   1 cup plain yogurt
>   1/8 cup vanilla protein powder
>   1/8 cup ground flax seeds
>   A few ice cubes

Mix together in blender. Makes about 2 servings.

Strawberry Banana Smoothie

>   1 cup fresh or frozen strawberries
>   1 banana
>   1/2 - 3/4 cup apple or white grape juice (more for thinner consistency)
>   1/8 cup protein powder
>   1 cup yogurt
>   1/8 cup ground flax seeds

Mix together in blender. Makes about 2 servings.

References

Aldercreutz, H. and Mazur, W.; Phytoestrogens and Western diseases. Ann. Med. 1997; 29:95.

Arjmandi, BH; Nutrition Research 1998 Jul; 18(7): 1203-14.

Arjmandi BH; The role of phytoestrogens in the prevention and treatment of osteoporosis in ovarian hormone deficiency. J Am Coll Nutr. 2001 Oct;20(5 Suppl):398S-402S; disc. 417S-420S. Review.

Axelson M, Sjövall J, Gustafsson BE, Setchell KDR.; Origin of lignans in mammals and identification of a precursor from plants. Nature 1982; 298: 659-660.

Beckman KB, Ames BN.; The free radical theory of aging matures, Physiol Rev. 1998 Apr;78(2):547-81. Review.

Bhathena SJ, Velasquez MT.. Beneficial role of dietary phytoestrogens in obesity and diabetes. Am. J. Clin. Nutr. 2002, 76: 1191-1201.

Bierenbaum ML, et al; Reducing atherogenic risk in hyperlipemic humans with flax seed supplementation: a preliminary report. J Am Coll Nutr 1993;12:501-4.

Brooks, J.; Ward,W.; et al Supplementation with flaxseed alters estrogen metabolism in postmenopausal women to a greater extent than does supplementation with an equal amount of soy. American Journal of Clinical Nutrition 2004; 79:318-325.

Chen J, et al; Dietary flaxseed enhances the inhibitory effect of tamoxifen on the growth of estrogen-dependent human breast cancer (mcf-7) in nude mice. Clin Cancer Res. 2004 Nov 15;10(22):7703-11.

Chen J, et al; Exposure to flaxseed or its purified lignan during suckling inhibits chemically induced rat mammary tumorigenesis. Exp Biol Med (Maywood) 2003 Sep;228(8):951-8.

Clark WF, Kortas C, et al; Flaxseed in lupus nephritis: a two-year nonplacebo-controlled crossover study. J Am Coll Nutr. 2001 Apr;20(2 Suppl):143-8.

Clark WF, Muir AD, Westcott ND, Parbtani A.; A novel treatment for lupus nephritis: lignan precursor derived from flax. Lupus. 2000;9(6):429-36.

Clark WF, Parbtani A, Huff MW,et al; Flaxseed: a potential treatment for lupus nephritis. Kidney Int 1995 Aug;48(2):475-80.

Cunnane S.C., et al; Nutritional attributes of traditional flaxseed in healthy young adults. Am J Clin Nutr. 1995 Jan;61(1):62-8.

Cunnane. S.C., et al.; Nutritional attributes of traditional flaxseed in healthy young adults. Amer. J. Clin. Nutr. 1992; 61:62.

Cunnane SC, Ganguli S, et al.; High alpha-linolenic acid flaxseed: some nutritional properties in humans. Department of Nutritional Sciences, Faculty of Medicine, University of Toronto, Canada. Br J Nutr 1993 Mar;69(2):443-53.

Das, U.N.: Anti-cancer effects of cis-unsaturated fatty acids both in vitro and invivo. In : Lipid-Soluble Antioxidants: Biochemistry and Clinical Applications. Ong. A.S.H. and Packer. L., eds. Basel/Switzerland: Birkhauser Verlag, 1992; 482.

Das, U.N. 1995. Tumoricidal action of gamma-linolenic acid with particular reference to the therapy of human glioma. Med. Sci. Res 23:507.

de Kleijn MJ, van der Schouw YT, Wilson PW, et al. Dietary intake of phytoestrogens is associated with a favorable metabolic cardiovascular risk profile in postmenopausal U.S.women: the Framingham study. J Nutr. 2002 Feb;132(2):276-82

DeMarco, D.M. et al.; Effects of fatty acids on proliferation and activation of human synovial compartment lymphocytes. J. Leukocyle Biol. 1994; 56:612.

Demark-Wahnefried W, Robertson CN, Walther PJ, Polascik TJ, Paulson DF, Vollmer RT; Pilot study to explore effects of low-fat, flaxseed-supplemented diet on proliferation of benign prostatic epithelium and prostate-specific antigen. Urology 2004 May;63(5):900-4.

Demark-Wahnefried W, et al; Pilot study of dietary fat restriction and flaxseed supplementation in men with prostate cancer before surgery: exploring the effects on hormonal levels, prostate-specific antigen, and histopathologic features. Duke University Medical Center, Urology 2001 Jul;58(1):47-52.

Denis L, Morton MS, Griffiths K.; Diet and its preventive role in prostatic disease Eur Urol. 1999;35(5-6):377-87.

De Stefani E et al Alpha-linolenic acid and risk of prostate cancer: a case control study in Uruguay. Cancer Epidemiol Biomarkers Prev 2000 Mar;9(3):335-8.

Dinkova-Kostova AT, Gang DR, Davin LB, et al. 1996. (+)-Pinoresinol/ (+)-lariciresinol reductase from Forsythia intermedia. J. Biol. Chem. 271: 29473-29482.

Dodin S, et al; The effects of flaxseed dietary supplement on lipid profile, bone mineral density, and symptoms in menopausal women: a randomized, double-blind, wheat germ placebo-controlled clinical trial. Clin Endocrinol Metab. 2005 Mar;90(3):1390-7.

Evans BA, et al; Inhibition of 5 alpha-reductase in genital skin fibroblasts and prostate tissue by dietary lignans and isoflavonoids. J Endocrinol. 1995 Nov;147(2):295-302.

Ford JD, et al; Biosynthetic pathway to the cancer chemopreventive secoisolariciresinol diglucoside-hydroxymethyl glutaryl ester-linked lignan oligomers in flax (Linum usitatissimum) seed. J Nat Prod. 2001 Nov;64(11):1388-97.

Franco OH, et al; Higher dietary intake of lignans is associated with better cognitive performance in postmenopausal women. J. Nutr. 2005 May, 135:1190-1195

Gann PH et al. Prospective Study of Plasma Fatty Acids and Risk of Prostate Cancer. Journal of the National Cancer Institute, Vol. 86, No. 4, February 16, 1994, p. 281-6.

Goss PE, Li T, Pinto S, Thompson LU; Effects of Dietary Flaxseed in Women with Cyclical Mastalgia. Breast Cancer Res Treat 2000; 64:49

Griffiths K, Denis L, Turkes A, Morton MS.; Phytoestrogens and diseases of the prostate gland. Baillieres Clin Endocrinol Metab. 1998 Dec;12(4):625-47. Review.

Haggans CJ, Hutchins AM, Olson BA, Thomas W, Martini MC, Slavin JL.; Effect of flaxseed consumption on urinary estrogen metabolites in postmenopausal women. Nutr Cancer 1999;33:188-195.

Haggans CJ, Travelli EJ, Thomas W, Martini MC, Slavin JL.; The effect of flaxseed and wheat bran consumption on urinary estrogen metabolites in premenopausal women. Cancer Epidemiol Biomarkers Prev. 2000 Jul;9(7):719-25.

Hall AV, Parbtani A, Clark WF, et al; Abrogation of MRL/lpr lupus nephritis by dietary flaxseed. Am J Kidney Dis. 1993 Aug;22(2):326-32.

Harris RK, Haggerty WJ. 1993. Assays for potentially anticarcinogenic phytochemicals in flaxseed. Cereal Foods World 38: 147-151. 26.

Harvei S et al. Prediagnostic Levels of Fatty Acids in Serum Phospholipids: n-3 and n-6 Fatty Acids and the Risk of Prostate Cancer. Inter. Journal of Cancer, 1997: 71; 545-51.

Hedelin M, et. al. Dietary phytoestrogen, serum enterolactone and risk of prostate cancer: the cancer prostate Sweden study (Sweden). Cancer Causes Control. 2006 Mar;17(2):169-80.

Hong SJ, Kim SI, Kwon SM, Lee JR,: Chung BC.; Comparative study of concentration of isoflavones and lignans in plasma and prostatic tissues of normal control and benign prostatic hyperplasia.Yonsei Med J 2002 Apr;43(2):236-41.

Hutchins AM, et al; Flaxseed consumption influences endogenous hormone concentrations in postmenopausal women. Nutr Cancer. 2001;39(1):58-65.

Hutchins AM, et el; Flaxseed influences urinary lignan excretion in a dose-dependent manner in postmenopausal women.Cancer Epidemiol Biomarkers Prev. 2000 Oct;9(10):1113-8.

Hutchins AM, Slavin JL.; Effects of flaxseed on sex hormone metabolism. In: Flaxseed in Human Nutrition, eds Thompson LU and Cunnane SC, 2nd ed, AOCS Press, 2003 Champaign, IL, pp. 126-149. 122.

Ingram, A.J., et al.; Effects of flaxseed and flax oil diets in a rat-5/6 renal ablation model. Amer. J. Kidney Dis. 1995; 25(2):320.

Ingram. D., et al.; Case-control study of phytoestrogens and breast cancer. Lancet 1997; 350(9083):990.

Jenab M. Thompson LU.;The influence of flaxseed and lignans on colon carcinogenesis and beta-glucuronidase activity. Carcinogenesis. 1996 Jun;17(6):1343-8.

Jenkins DJ, et al; Health aspects of partially defatted flaxseed, including effects on serum lipids, oxidative measures, and ex vivo androgen and progestin activity: a controlled crossover trial. Am J Clin Nutr. 1999 Mar;69(3):395-402.

Kirkman LM, Lampe JW, Campbell DR, et al.; Urinary lignan and isoflavonoid excretion in men and women consuming vegetable and soy diets. Nutr. Cancer 1995. 24: 1-12.

Kitts DD, et al; Antioxidant activity of the flaxseed lignan secoisolariciresinol diglycoside and its mammalian lignan metabolites enterodiol/enterolactone. Mol. Cell. Biochem. 1999; 202: 91-100.

Knight. D.C. and Eden. J.A.. A review of the clinical effects of phytoestrogens. Obstet. Gynecol. 1996; 87:897.

Kreijkamp-Kaspers S, Kok L, Bots ML, Grobbee DE, van der Schouw YT.; Dietary phytoestrogens and vascular function in postmenopausal women: a cross-sectional study. J Hypertens. 2004 Jul;22(7):1381-8.

Kuijsten A, et al; Pharmacokinetics of enterolignans in health men and women consuming a single dose of secoisolariciresinol diglucoside. J. Nutr. 2005 Apr, 135:795-801.

Lemay A, et al; 2002. Flaxseed dietary supplement versus hormone replacement therapy in hypercholesterolemic menopausal women. Obstet. Gynecol. 100: 495-504.

Lampe, J.W.; Urinary lignan and isoflavonoid excretion in premenopausal women consuming flaxseed powder. Am J Clin Nutr 60: 122-128.

Lei B, Roncaglia V, Vigano R, Cremonini C, et al; Phytoestrogens and liver disease. Mol Cell Endocrinol. 2002 Jul 31;193(1-2):81.

Lemay, A ,et al; Flaxseed Dietary Supplement Versus Hormone Replacement Therapy in hypercholesterolemic Menopausal Women. Obstetrics & Gynecology 2002;100:495-504.

Levander, O.A. et al;Antimalarial effects of flaxseed and flaxseed oil. In: Flaxseed in Human Nutrition, ed. S.C. Cunnane and L.U. Thompson. Champaign, IL: AOCS Press, 1995; 237-243.

Lin X, Switzer BR, Demark-Wahnefried W.; Effect of mammalian lignans on the growth of prostate cancer cell lines. Division of Urologic Surgery, Duke University Medical Center, Durham, NC. Anticancer Res 2001 Nov-Dec;21(6A):3995-9.

Lin X, Gingrich JR, Bao W, Li J, Haroon ZA, Demark-Wahnefried W.; Effect of flaxseed supplementation on prostatic carcinoma in transgenic mice. Urology 2002 May;60(5):919-24.

Lucas EA, Wild RD, et al; Flaxseed improves lipid profile without altering biomarkers of bone metabolism in postmenopausal women. Department of Nutritional Sciences, Oklahoma State University, J Clin Endocrinol Metab 2002 Apr;87(4):1527-32.

Madhavi, N., et al.; Supression of human T-cell growth in vitro by cis-unsaturated faty acids: relationship to free radicals and lipid peroxidation. Prostagland. Leukolri. Ess. Fatty Acids 1994; 51:33.

Mantzioris, E. MJ James, RA Gibson, and LG Cleland, Nutritional attributes of dietary flaxseed oil. Am J Clin Nutr 1995 62: 841-842.

Marlett JA, et al; American Dietetic Association. Position of the American Dietetic Association: health implications of dietary fiber.J Am Diet Assoc 2002 Jul;102(7):993-1000.

McCann MJ.; Role of mammalian lignans in the prevention and treatment of prostate cancer. Nutr Cancer. 2005;52(1):1-14.

Milder IE, Arts IC, van de Putte B, Venema DP, Hollman PC. Lignan contents of Dutch plant foods: a database including lariciresinol, pinoresinol, secoisolariciresinol and matairesinol. Br J Nutr. 2005;93(3):393-402.

Morrissey C, Watson RW.; Phytoestrogens and prostate cancer; Curr Drug Targets. 2003 Apr;4(3):231-41.

Morton MS, et al; Determination of lignans and isoflavonoids in human female plasma following dietary supplementation. J. Endocrinol.1994. 142: 251-259.

Morton MS, Matos-Ferreira A, Abranches-Monteiro L, Correia R, Blacklock N, Chan PS, Cheng C, Lloyd S, Chieh-ping W, Griffiths K.; Measurement and metabolism of isoflavonoids and lignans in the human male. Cancer Lett. 1997 Mar 19;114(1-2):145-51

Muir AD, Westcott ND, Quantitation of the lignan secoisolariciresinol diglucoside in baked goods containing flax seed or flax meal. J Agric Food Chem. 2000 Sep;48(9):4048-52.

Nielsen SE, Freese R, Kleemola P, Mutanen M. 2002. Flavonoids in human urine as biomarkers for intake of fruits and vegetables. Cancer Epidemiol. Biomarkers Prev. 11: 459-466.

Nesbitt, P.D., Yi Lam, Thompson L.; Human metabolism of mammalian lignan precursors in raw and processed flaxseed. Am J Clin Nutr. 1999 69: 549-555.

Olson JA, Kobayashi S.; Antioxidants in health and disease: overview. Proc Soc Exp Biol Med. 1992 Jun;200(2):245-7. Review.

Oomah BD, et al.1998. Flaxseed products for disease prevention. In: Functional Foods: Biochemical & Processing Aspects, ed Mazza G, Technomic Publishing, Lancaster, PA; 91-138.

Oomah BD, et al. 1995. Phenolic acids in flaxseed. J. Agric. Food Chem. 43: 2016-2019.

Orcheson LJ, Rickard SE, Seidl MM, Thompson LU; Flaxseed and its mammalian lignan precursor cause a lengthening or cessation of estrous cycling in rats. Cancer Lett. 1998 Mar 13;125(1-2):69-76

Pattanaik U, Prasad K.; Oxygen Free Radicals and Endotoxic Shock: Effect of Flaxseed. J Cardiovasc Pharmacol Ther. 1998 Oct;3(4):305-318.

Peat, R. Ray Peat's Newsletter, 1997 Issue, pg 3.

Phipps WR, Martini MC, Lampe JW, et al. 1993. Effect of flax seed ingestion on the menstrual cycle. J. Clin. Endocrinol. Metab. 1998. 77: 1215-1219.

Prasad K.; Secoisolariciresinol diglucoside from flaxseed delays the development of type 2 diabetes in Zucker rat. J Lab Clin Med. 2001 Jul;138(1):32-9.

Prasad K.; Oxidative stress as a mechanism of diabetes in diabetic BB prone rats: effect of secoisolariciresinol diglucoside (SDG). Mol Cell Biochem. 2000 Jun;209(1-2):89-96.

Prasad K, et al; Protective effect of secoisolariciresinol diglucoside against streptozotocin-induced diabetes and its mechanism. Mol Cell Biochem. 2000 Mar;206(1-2):141-9

Prasad K.; Flaxseed: a source of hypocholesterolemic and antiatherogenic agents, Drug News Perspect 2000 Mar;13(2):99-

Prasad K.; Reduction of serum cholesterol and hypercholesterolemic atherosclerosis in rabbits by secoisolariciresinol diglucoside isolated from flaxseed. Circulation 1999 Mar 16;99(10):1355-62

Prasad K, Mantha SV, Muir AD, Westcott ND.; Reduction of hypercholesterolemic atherosclerosis by CDC-flaxseed with very low alpha-linolenic acid. Atherosclerosis 1998 Feb;136(2):367-75.

Prasad K.; Hydroxyl radical-scavenging property of secoisolariciresinol diglucoside (SDG) isolated from flax-seed. Mol. Cell. Biochem. 1997,168: 117-123.

Prasad K; Hypocholesterolemic and antiatherosclerotic effect of flax lignan complex isolated from flaxseed. Atherosclerosis 2005 Apr, 179(2):269-275.

Praticò D.; In vivomeasurement of the redox state. Lipids 2001 36: S45-S47.

Ramanathan, R., et al.; Effects of Gamma-linolenic acid, flavonoids, and vitamins on cytotoxicity and lipid peroxidation. Free Rod. Biol. Med. 1994;16:43.

Rickard SE, et al, Plasma insulin-like growth factor I levels in rats are reduced by dietary supplementation of flaxseed or its lignan secoisolariciresinol diglycoside. Cancer Lett. 2000 Dec 8;161(1):47-55.

Rickard SE, Yuan YV, Chen J, Thompson LU; Dose effects of flaxseed and its lignan on N-methyl-N-nitrosourea-induced mammary tumorigenesis in rats. Nutr Cancer 1999;35(1):50-7.

Rickard SE, Thompson LU.; Phytoestrogens and lignans: Effects on reproduction and chronic disease. In: Antinutrients and Phytochemicals in Foods, ed Shahidi F, Oxford University Press, 1997, New York, pp. 273-293.

Ridges L, Sunderland R, Moerman K, Meyer B, Astheimer L, Howe P.; Cholesterol lowering benefits of soy and linseed enriched foods. Asia Pac J Clin Nutr. 2001;10(3):204-11.

Rickard, S.E. Health effects of flaxseed mucilage, lignans. INFORM 1997. 8(8):860.

Sano T, Oda E, et al; Antithrombic and anti-atherogenic effects of partially defatted flaxseed meal using a laser-induced thrombosis test in apolipoprotein E and low-density lipoprotein receptor deficient mice. Blood Coagul Fibrinolysis 2003 Dec; 14(8):707-12.

Simopoulos A, Am J Clin Nutr, 70 (3 Suppl) 1999.

Stattin P, Adlercreutz H, et al; Circulating enterolactone and prostate cancer risk: a Nordic nested case-control study. Int J Cancer. 2002 May 1;99(1):124-9.

Sung MK, Lautens M, Thompson LU. Mammalian lignans inhibit the growth of estrogen-independent human colon tumor cells. Anticancer Res. 1998 May-Jun;18(3A):1405-8.

Tan KP, et al; Mammary gland morphogenesis is enhanced by exposure to flaxseed or its major lignan during suckling in rats. Exp Biol Med (Maywood) 2004;229(2):147-57.

Tham DM, et al; Potential health benefits of dietary phytoestrogens: A review of the clinical, epidemiological, and mechanistic evidence. J. Clin. Endocrinol. Metab. 1998, 83: 2223-2235.

Thompson, L, Cunnane, S.; Flaxseed in Human Nutrition, AOCS Press, Champaign, IL, 1995; Chapter 10 Flaxseed and Glucose Metabolism by Thomas MS. Wolever.

Thompson, L.U.. et al.; Flaxseed and its lignan and oil compo?nents reduce mammary tumour growth at a late stage of Carcinogenesis 1997.17 (6):13.

Thompson LU, Seidl MM, Rickard SE, Orcheson LJ, Fong HH; Antitumorigenic effect of a mammalian lignan precursor from flaxseed. Nutr Cancer 1996; 26(2):159-65

Thompson LU, Rickard SE, Cheung F, et al. 1997. Variability in anticancer lignan levels in flaxseed. Nutr. Cancer 27: 26-30.

Thompson LU, et al; Dietary flaxseed alter tumor biological markers in postmenopausal breast cancer. Clin. Cancer Research 2005 May, 11:3828-3835

Thompson LU. 2003. Analysis and bioavailability of lignans. In: Flaxseed in Human Nutrition, eds Thompson LU and Cunnane SC, 2nd ed, AOCS Press, Champaign, IL, pp. 92-116.

Tou JC, et al;Exposure to flaxseed or its lignan component during different developmental stages influences rat mammary gland structures. Carcinogenesis 1999 Sep;20(9): 1831-5.

Triboulot C, et al; Dietary (n-3) polyunsaturated fatty acids exert antihypertensive effects by modulating calcium signaling in Tcells of rats. J Nutr. 2001 Sep;131(9):2364-9.

Usui T. Pharmaceutical prospects of phytoestrogens. Endocr J. 2006 Feb;53(1):7-20.

Van de Poll, L.; Phytoestrogens: health benefits, bioavailability and safety. Functional Foods, Nov/Dec. 2005.

van der Schouw YT, Pijpe A,etal; Higher usual dietary intake of phytoestrogens is associated with lower aortic stiffness in postmenopausal women. Arterioscler Thromb Vasc Biol. 2002 Aug 1;22(8):1316-22.

van der Schouw YT, et al; The usual intake of lignans but not that of isoflavones may be related to cardiovascular risk factors in U.S. men. J Nutr. 2005 Feb;135(2):260-6.

van der Schouw YT, et al; Prospective study on usual dietary phytoestrogen intake and cardiovascular disease risk in Western women. Circulation. 2005 Feb 1;111(4):465-71.

Vanharanta M, et al.; Association between low serum enterolactone and increased plasma F2-isoprostanes, a measure of lipid peroxidation. J Nutr. 2002 Feb;132(2):276-82.

Vanharanta M, Voutilainen S, Rissanen TH, et al.; Risk of cardiovascular disease-related and all-cause death according to serum concentrations of enterolactone: Kuopio Ischaemic Heart Disease Risk Factor Study. Arch Intern Med. 2003 May 12;163(9):1099-104.

Vanharanta M, Voutilainen S, et al; Risk of acute coronary events according to serum concentrations of enterolactone: a prospective population-based case-control study. Lancet. 1999 Dec 18-25;354(9196):2112-5.

Velicer, C, et al.; Antibiotic Use Linked to Breast Cancer Risk? Journal of the American Medical Association, February 18, 2004

Vijay Kumar, K. and Das. U.N.; Lipid peroxides and essential fatty acids in patients with doronary heart disease. J. Nutr. Med. 1994; 4(1):33.

Wang L.; Mammalian phytoestrogens: enterodiol and enterolactone. J Chromatogr B Analyt Technol Biomed Life Sci. 2002 Sep 25;777(1-2):289.

Wang LQ, Meselhy MR, Li Y, Qin GW, Hattori M.; Human intestinal bacteria capable of transforming secoisolariciresinol diglucoside to mammalian lignans, enterodiol and enterolactone. Chem Pharm Bull (Tokyo). 2000 Nov;48(11):1606-10.

Wang L, Chen J, Thompson LU. The inhibitory effect of flaxseed on the growth and metastasisof estrogen receptor negative human breast cancer xenograftsis attributed to both its lignan and oil components. Int J Cancer.2005 Apr 22;

Ward WE, Jiang FO, Thompson LU; Exposure to flaxseed or purified lignan during lactation influences rat mammary gland structures. Nutr Cancer 2000;37(2):187-92.

Westcott ND, Muir AD.;Flax lignan update. Saskatchewan Flax Grower 2003,4: 6.

Wilcox G, Wahlqvist ML, Burger HG, Medley G. 1990. Oestrogenic effects of plant foods in postmenopausal women. Br. Med. J. 301: 905-906.

ABOUT THE AUTHORS

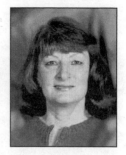

Irene H. Sönju lived the first seven years of her life in the rich Red River Valley Region of North Dakota, where her father planted flax seed as the highest paying cash crop in the fifties. Two years after her fathers passing in 1955, she moved to a small farm with her mother, step-father, and seven brothers and sisters in the Ottertail Lake region of Minnesota. Irene is knowledgeable about growing grains and livestock. She knows the importance of soil type and semi arid climate conditions for growing flax with high nutritional value. She helped gather in the harvest fields; loved roaming the woods and swamps, swimming in Ottertail Lake; and invested in livestock.

Irene is back to her country roots and love of the land through her involvement in writing, speaking and educating the public on the health benefits of flax seed and SDG lignans.

Irene H. Sönju lives in Kandiyohi County, "where the lakes begin". She is a Former Sotheby's Associate as an Art Dealer for Emerging Artists. For over twenty-five years she has enjoyed collecting Original Art. Irene has a BA degree from St. John's University/College of St. Benedict where she majored in Art History and Studio Art.

Contact: Irene H. Sönju, Willmar,MN. 1-877-544-6267 or (320) 235-7249
Email: ihsonju@yahoo.com

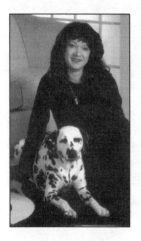

Beth M. Ley, Ph.D., has been a science writer specializing in health and nutrition since 1988 and has written many health-related books, including the best sellers, **DHEA: Unlocking the Secrets to the Fountain of Youth** and **MSM: On Our Way Back to Health With Sulfur**. She wrote her own undergraduate degree program and graduated in Scientific and Technical Writing from North Dakota State University in 1987 (combination of Zoology and Journalism). Dr. Beth has her masters (1998) and doctoral degrees (1999) in Nutrition.

Dr. Beth does Biblical-based nutrition and wellness counseling in Golden Valley, MN, (Twin Cities Area) and also on line (www.blpublications.com). She speaks on Biblical nutrition, health and Divine healing locally and nationwide.

Beth (also a ND native) currently lives in the Minneapolis area. She is dedicated to God and to spreading the health message. She enjoys nature and spending time with her dalmation, KC.

Memberships: American Academy of Anti-aging, New York Academy of Sciences, Oxygen Society and Resurrection Apostolic International Network (RAIN),

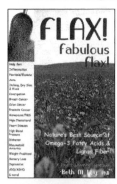
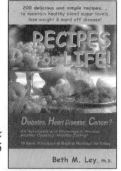
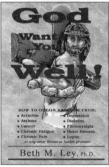
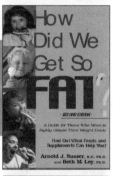
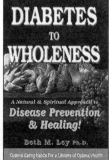
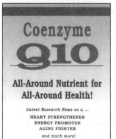
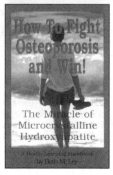

TO PLACE AN ORDER:

——	***Aspirin Alternatives: The Top Natural Pain-Relieving Analgesics*** (Lombardi)	$8.95
——	***Bilberry & Lutein: The Vision Enhancers!*** (Ley)	$4.95
——	***Calcium: The Facts, Fossilized Coral*** (Ley)	$4.95
——	***Castor Oil: Its Healing Properties*** (Ley)	$3.95
——	***Dr. John Willard on Catalyst Altered Water*** (Ley)	$3.95
——	***Chlorella: Ultimate Green Food (Ley)***	$4.95
——	***CoQ10: All-Around Nutrient for All-Around Health*** (Ley)	$4.95
——	***Colostrum: Nature's Gift to the Immune System*** (Ley)	$5.95
——	***DHA: The Magnificent Marine Oil*** (Ley)	$6.95
——	***DHEA: Unlocking the Secrets/Fountain of Youth-2nd ed.*** (Ash & Ley) . . .	$14.95
——	***Diabetes to Wholeness*** (Ley)	$9.95
——	***Discover the Beta Glucan Secret*** (Ley)	$3.95
——	***Fading: One family's journey ... Alzheimer's*** (Kraft)	$12.95
——	***Flax! Fabulous Flax!*** (Ley)	$4.95
——	***Flax Lignans: Fifty Years to Harvest*** (Sönju & Ley)	$4.95
——	***God Wants You Well*** (Ley)	$14.95
——	***Health Benefits of Probiotics*** (Dash)	$4.95
——	***How Did We Get So Fat? 2nd Edition*** (Susser & Ley)	$8.95
——	***How to Fight Osteoporosis and Win!*** (Ley)	$6.95
——	***Maca: Adaptogen and Hormone Balancer (Ley)***	$4.95
——	***Marvelous Memory Boosters*** (Ley)	$3.95
——	***Medicinal Mushrooms:*** Agaricus Blazei Murill *(Ley)*	$4.95
——	***MSM: On Our Way Back to Health W/ Sulfur*** (Ley) SPANISH	$3.95
——	***MSM: On Our Way Back to Health W/ Sulfur*** (Ley)	$4.95
——	***Natural Healing Handbook*** (Ley)	$14.95
——	***Nature's Road to Recovery: Nutritional Supplements for the Alcoholic & Chemical Dependent*** (Ley)	$5.95
——	***PhytoNutrients: Medicinal Nutrients in Foods***, Revised /Updated (Ley) .	$5.95
——	***Recipes For Life! (Spiral Bound Cookbook)*** (Ley)	$19.95
——	***Secrets the Oil Companies Don't Want You to Know*** (LaPointe) . . .	$10.00
——	***Spewed! How to Cast Out Lukewarm Christianity through Fasting and a Fasted Lifestyle -***	$15.95
——	***The Potato Antioxidant: Alpha Lipoic Acid*** (Ley)	$6.95
——	***Vinpocetine: Revitalize Your Brain w/ Periwinkle Extract!*** (Ley)	$4.95

Book subtotal $ _____ + $5.00 shipping = $ _____

Send check or money order to:
BL Publications 649 Kayla Lane, Hanover, MN 55341

Credit card orders please call toll free: 1-877-BOOKS11
For more info visit: www.blpublications.com